Table of Contents

Understanding and Managing Allergy-Related Coughs

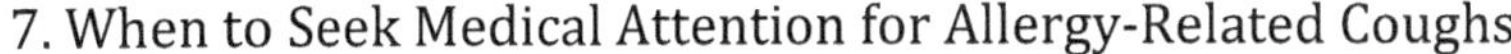

Comprehensive Guide to Allergy Cough: Symptoms, Treatment Options, and More

1. Introduction to Allergy Cough

What is allergy cough? Let's start by understanding what an allergy cough or cough-variant asthma (CVA) is. An allergy cough presents itself as dry, persistent coughing and is often accompanied by postnasal drip. The cough, in this case, is simply the body's normal response to the inflammation of the airway and the production of too much saliva. Meanwhile, postnasal drip can occur when the mucus from the sinuses enters the throat. It has a thin consistency (unlike the thick mucus that comes up with a cold) and is usually clear in color. The combination of these two can hence lead one to cough. It is essential to have a good understanding of the kind of cough that you are dealing with, as an appropriate approach to treatment can ensure that you can get relief in a shorter span of time. In this definitive guide to allergy cough, we seek to enlighten our readers about measures to reduce exposure to irritants and prevent an allergy cough, diagnostic procedures and tests for allergy cough, and available treatments for allergy cough. Do continue reading!

Let's talk about allergy cough first. Presently, more and more people suffer from seasonal or year-round allergies. But, do you know that allergies can also cause a chronic cough? In this comprehensive guide to allergy cough, we discuss all you need to know about this specific type of cough. We cover everything about allergy-induced cough, ranging from its symptoms, diagnostic procedure, treatment options, and many more. Keep on reading to learn about the link between allergy and cough!

2. Understanding Allergies and Coughing

In a person with allergies, the immune system might mistakenly identify foreign substances as harmful. These substances can range from certain foods to environmental triggers such as dust mites, pet dander, and grass pollen. When allergens enter the body, an overactive immune response occurs. This response leads to the wider release of a signaling chemical (histamine) that marks other cells as harmful agents. This, in turn, leads to a chain reaction that can extend to the respiratory system and cause coughing. Coughing can often be the result of symptoms stemming from allergies, and determining the right treatment, preventive measures, and management techniques necessitates understanding the underlying cause of the coughing. Coughing during allergic reactions is essentially the body's way of clearing the respiratory passages of extra mucus, particles, and irritants caused by an exposed allergen.

Allergic cough, also known as allergy cough, is a common health condition characterized by coughing that may worsen depending on exposure to given triggers or allergens. When someone suffering from an allergy is exposed to the responsible allergen, their body mounts a series of defense responses. These responses result in the release of a chemical compound called histamine that triggers inflammatory responses and can lead to mucus formation, nasal congestion, irritated airways, and subsequently, coughing. Symptoms can range from mild to severe, and allergy coughing can either be acute, lasting less than 8 weeks, or chronic, exceeding 8 weeks. To successfully treat allergy cough, patients should first understand some key aspects of the relationship between allergies and coughing.

3. Common Allergens that Trigger Coughing

If you have an allergy-induced cough, the allergens that may be causing it are called triggers. Numerous substances in the environment can trigger the release of histamine and other chemicals in your body, causing coughing. Knowing which substances are potential triggers can help you manage your exposure and learn how to cope with your allergy cough.

- Pollens: Pollen grains are released from plants (flowering plants, grasses, and weeds) that cause allergic rhinitis and conjunctivitis (hay fever). In some cases, these pollens may lead to contributing to asthma. - Dust Mites: Dust mites are microscopic organisms that live in beddings, mattresses, upholstered furniture, and carpets. The remnants that dust mites leave behind can cause inhalant allergies. - Molds: Outdoor molds occur in consistently moist areas like falling leaves, rotten wood, and grassy and grain areas. Indoor molds are mainly responsible for the growth of mold in areas where water damage or excessive moisture introduces growth, like in basements. - Cockroach allergens: When cockroaches die, their body parts and feces become airborne substances that trigger allergic reactions, especially for those who have asthma and allergies with eel gender-made proteins. - Animal dander: Protein is shed by cats, dogs, birds, and other household pets. Dead skin cells, hair, and secretions may serve as transporters. In sensitive individuals, these proteins cause respiratory allergic diseases.

Allergens are substances that can cause allergic reactions. Once a person encounters an allergen, an abnormal reaction from the immune system may occur, causing cough episodes. Allergen exposure in people with chronic cough (from allergic rhinitis or asthma, for example) leads to the release of airway mediators and nerve circuitry, which is an essential cause of coughing. Here are some common allergens that are responsible for causing coughing:

4. Symptoms of Allergy-Induced Cough

The first thing to remember is that some of the primary symptoms of coughing and allergies are really similar. As a result, it is strongly encouraged to see a licensed doctor if you have symptoms. Certain health agents, including common pollutants or scents, can cause a cough to occur in the short term. It is also possible to experience a short-term cough episode when a train, city bus, or any other type of transport pulls away. Having a doctor conduct an allergy exam or the newly available adverse allergy test can be beneficial. Unauthorized control and treatment can introduce additional health concerns, thus further testing is important. One of the first steps in asthma and allergies prevention and treatment is to get an allergic or environmental condition.

- Dripping or running nose - Eye-related symptoms such as itching, tearing, or dryness - Being triggered by excess allergens is a symptom of chronic cough. - A scratchy throat - Sinusitis - Nasal congestion - Wheezing - Labored breathing - Shortness of breath

Symptoms of cough in the presence of allergies are generally characterized by typical allergy symptoms, including nasal congestion, sneezing, sinus pain, and runny noses. These symptoms increase the likelihood that an allergy may be the cause of your cough.

5. Diagnosis of Allergy Cough

These tests check for specific immunoglobulin E (IgE) antibodies to allergens. Percent-predicted spirometry - Along with spirometry tests at rest, certain methods have been adapted to assess breathing limitations using a handheld spirometer device when measured at rest and after a bronchodilator challenge. Thoracic imaging, including chest x-rays - May be ordered to look for immune-related edemas as a potential cause of cough. Methacholine challenge (inhalational challenge testing) - This test is used in investigation allergy cough and asthma and tests for the degree of breathing airway hyperactivity. During testing, airborne treatments such as a saline placebo or methacholine are given in increasing concentrations while the patient breathes through a small respiratory device. Eucapnic voluntary hyperpnea (EVH) - Is useful for diagnosing exercise-induced bronchospasm based on bronchoprovocation testing induced by hyperpnea or breathing dry air. Currently, is the only method of testing for exercise-induced bronchoconstriction (EIB), but EVH is also an option.

Allergy testing - This is sometimes ordered to confirm whether you have allergic rhinitis and might need allergy programs. Skin prick tests are done in healthcare providers' offices, and food challenges and other tests can be ordered. In vitro blood tests - There are many types of these tests, and they are used rather than skin tests if you are unable to have skin testing for health reasons or are taking medications that can interfere with testing.

When you visit a healthcare provider to determine if you have allergy cough, the visit typically includes a health history review and a physical exam. In such appointments, healthcare professionals will inquire about the onset and duration of your symptoms and whether anything seems to trigger or worsen your coughing. They will also inquire about other symptoms such as sneezing, itching, runny nose, and postnasal drip. This information, along with the physical exam assessing your head, neck, throat, and lungs along with an examination of other body systems, can help determine whether your cough is likely to be caused by allergy.

Diagnosing Allergy Cough

6. Treatment Options for Allergy Cough

Immunotherapy: For allergic coughing! Allergens are numerous, each potent enough to trigger coughing fits. Though specific medications can get you some relief, your physician may also suggest dilution of allergen vials that are subcutaneously injected as a treatment called immunotherapy. The allergen extracts consist of active components from the plant, including house dust mites, cat dander, dog dander, and pollens. These allergen extracts are used to reduce the level of IgE-mediated activities. They ultimately reduce the level of inflammation and thus stabilize the immune response. Immunotherapy is prescribed to patients suffering from a runny nose or sneezing, which includes allergy-induced cough as well. Omalizumab is an anti-IgE therapy that has worked well in terms of efficacy.

Home remedies: A tried and true practice. If home remedies help in curing an ailment, then why opt for other options? Given that aloe vera or neem toothpaste helps preserve the tissues of the gums, certainly, a nutritional diet combined with warm honey did not cause any harm either. Honey taken along with warm water has proven effective in curing coughing as it reduces throat irritation. Steam therapy is another home remedy conducted by inhaling steam. This helps to release any nasal congestion and cures cough. Resting is a good therapy when it comes to any ailment. Don't exert extra pressure on your body when you fall ill. The body needs rest when an individual receives any form of a jab or suffers from a disease or infection. Get a great sleep, and you're feeling a sense of relaxation. So make sure to get proper sleep to get rid of allergy-induced cough.

Lifestyle modifications: Control first, cure later. These are the basic health habits that might change the path of an allergy-induced cough to take. Health habits often affect the body's response. So why not choose the best health habits to stay fit? Well, the first one is a proper diet schedule and the second is regular exercise of at least 30 minutes a day. Both these factors play a crucial role in the immune response. Furthermore, maintaining a hygienic environment may reduce the level of allergen build-up at your home. This may at least give you relief from allergy over a certain period of time.

Anti-allergy medications: Route to relief by blocking the response of the immune system to the allergen. These medications include antihistamines (Olopatadine), decongestants (Phenylephrine), and anticholinergics (Ipratropium bromide). Antihistamine blockers like Olopatadine work great to cure an allergy-induced cough activated by post-nasal drip. Olopatadine works to block the release of histamines.

6.1. Medications for Allergy Cough

Pholcodine is a cough suppressant that works by blocking nerve signals to the cough center in the brain. It can be given in syrup form to help soothe dry, scabbing coughs. Sometimes combined with decongestants, expectorants, and antihistamines, and can be found in OTC combination medications. Some OTC combination medications containing pholcodine (especially ones containing pseudoephedrine) can be located behind the store counter, and the quantity purchases may be restricted. Be sure to read the pholcodine product's drug label to determine if pholcodine is present. While these medications can be used to effectively treat allergy cough, doctors will work with each individual to decide which medication is best suited for treating the cough. Healthcare providers can also weigh the potential dangers and advantages of each medication for use in children, as well as the type and cause of the allergy that causes the cough.

Medications used to treat a cough caused by allergies (such as hay fever) are called cough suppressants or antitussives. The dextromethorphan (DXM) (Delsym) may be used to decrease the cough reflex and act on the cough center in the brain. It is usually sold over-the-counter (OTC) and is available in the form of liquids, lozenges, quick-dissolve strips, and granules. The most common side effects of dextromethorphan are dizziness, drowsiness, and stomach upset. Guaifenesin (also known as Mucinex and Robitussin) is an expectorant used to treat coughs. It works by breaking down and thinning mucus to help clear a congested and dragging cough. This medication comes in the form of OTC and prescription liquids, tablets, and extended-release tablets. Side effects of guaifenesin are uncommon, but they may include upset stomach.

1. Medications for Allergy Cough

Allergy Cough Treatments

6.2. Lifestyle Changes and Home Remedies

In addition to these measures, some home-based remedies can act as an auxiliary in the reduction of allergy cough. Eucalyptus, honey, tea, orange, and onion are the main ones, being very indicated not only to contribute to the control of coughing problems but also by improving the discomfort provoked by the symptoms.

- Reduce exposure to allergens: Reducing the exposure of allergens in the environments where the individual circulates is essential, especially at home. It is important to avoid leaving the windows open to make possible the entry of dust and other particles. On the contrary, it is interesting to opt for environments with air conditioning and to replace filters regularly. It is also advised to leave the shoes used on the street outside the house or, when entering with them, clean them very well to avoid bringing particles home. - Avoid smoking: Quitting smoking is also essential for the therapeutic management of allergy cough since tobacco smoke is a powerful allergen creator. - Special cleaning: It is interesting to clean the house frequently, especially sweeping, which can make the particles fly and, instead of leaving the house, make them stay in suspension in the environment. In addition, regular cleaning using a vacuum cleaner and wet cloths can keep the presence of allergens under control. All clothing should also be washed regularly to get rid of pet hair and other particles.

Many lifestyle modifications and home-based remedies can complement drug treatments for cough caused by allergies.

Some habits can help a lot in keeping the condition always under control and, consequently, avoiding the discomfort promoted by the cough. Some of them include:

6.3. Immunotherapy for Allergy-Induced Cough

Indications: Patients who experience obstruction in daily life after avoiding allergens, people allergic to only 1 or a few antigens, asthma, and/or allergic rhinitis patients who receive inadequate relief from avoiding allergens, medications must be taken daily, and people who are consistently exposed to frequent triggers. The Principle: "What Caused the Allergy (IgE-Reactive Antigen)", "Controlling the Symptoms That Can Cause the Allergy (Immediate and Delayed Phase Chronic Care)", and "What Damage and Side Effects May Occur (Risk of Adverse Effects and Their Control)" are the three general principles of allergy treatment (Potential Benefits). Local symptoms: Slight redness after the injection (it will resolve on its own). Potential Benefits: Asthma and rhinitis control, decreased symptoms and prognosis, reduced incidence of new allergens, reduced need for other medications. Considering the Principles and the Treatment of Allergy Cough, the Approaches to Allergy Cough: What to Do When You Cannot Avoid Allergens, What Is the Benefit and Principle of Immunotherapy? PT Arindo Yogyakarta Sutrisnono, 2014.

Immunotherapy is a targeted treatment approach aimed at specific allergens. Since it's a medication and not a cure, the first step is to avoid what triggers your condition. Furthermore, it is essential to determine the roles of immunotherapy when making a personalized care plan. Then, immunotherapy may be suitable for patients who give their consent after the advantages and risks have been fully explained. Immunotherapy may occasionally be added to the treatment plan for patients who do not respond to or who dislike taking corticosteroid drugs on a regular basis. Allergic cough can be caused by a variety of factors. Thus, since it is poorly affected by general cough medicine treatment, a specialized approach is required. A patient with a cough for an extended period could have an allergy cough. The cough is caused by a person's immune system overreacting to allergy-causing substances in the air (allergens).

7. Prevention Strategies for Allergy Cough

- Dust often. This involves vacuuming floors and furniture. Make sure to use a vacuum cleaner with a HEPA filter. Wash all bedding once a week in hot water. - Cover pillows and mattresses. To avoid dust mites from getting in, use a cover that is dust-mite resistant. - Eliminate clutter. Anything that collects dust, such as knick-knacks, books, and magazines, should be removed from your home. - Plants: To keep dust under control, use only plants that cleanse the air. - You don't have to help an allergy cough by letting your lawn grip thick with pollen. When pollen levels are greatest, staying indoors can help you avoid inhaling it. Keep your windows shut and use an air conditioner if at all feasible. In the middle of the day, keep your windows closed during peak pollen seasons.

To keep your home more allergen-free, make a few extra adjustments. Breathing in warm, damp air makes allergy coughing worse. Use the bathroom fan or keep a window open to keep the room dry.

Ingesting trigger foods can also cause an allergy cough. Talk to your doctor to avoid them.

Because an allergy cough is most often induced by inhaling irritants such as pet dander, pollen, and dust mites, preventing contact with these allergens is the best way to protect yourself. Follow the steps below to reduce your exposure to allergens and thus decrease your risk of developing an allergy cough.

8. Managing Allergy Cough in Different Age Groups

Typically, acute rhinitis (AR) of either allergic and viral etiology in children results in a middle ear effusion that can frequently become chronic and produce obstructive complications. Middle ear organ damage (OMD) occurs in early childhood in the upper eustachian tube (ETEar) due to the summation of risk factors resulting in ET quantum engine dysfunction matrix and ventilation organ failure (VOF) resulting in the common ear pressure changes from a non-dysfunctional mucous adhesion effect. In adults, these OMD are seen as more fibrosis induced by inflammation leading to a decrease in patency. In both cases, the hearing loss caused can significantly affect QoL, especially in aging. Management requires synonymous AR and OME control to regain good QoL. This guide will address the considerations for managing an AR-cough for different age periods in life.

In contrast, within the adult population, there is a growing interest in the proven impact of anti-IL-5 therapy on the upper eustachian tube blockage (ETEar) as reflected in reduced OME symptoms data correlating with decreased blood and tissue eosinophils. The elderly may experience a faster degradation and/or half-life of certain medications, have multiple medication therapies to manage, or are affected by age-associated comorbidities or frailty, influencing their ability to perform an optimized self-care for their AR.

Managing an allergy cough may require different considerations based on an individual's age and natural history. One study found that allergic rhinitis represented a significant pediatric health issue, but it is often underdiagnosed and consequently undertreated. Paradoxically, when studied, it was found that the most commonly used medication in children with AR were antihistamines, followed by inhaled glucocorticoids and antileukotrienes. While long-term pharmacotherapy is often efficacious, age-specific guidelines will take into account the clinician's experience, the severity of the symptoms, and the persistence and exacerbation pattern of AR. Therefore, adherence and patient-centered endpoints, including those of QoL, should be achieved in such patients.

8.1. Children and Allergy Cough

Indoor allergies for children are mostly allergens from their immediate living environment. Children with allergies cough when exposed to house dust, mites, cockroaches, fungi, paint smells, animals such as cats and dogs, and secondhand smoke. Food allergies can make some children cough, but these involve various changes in the gastrointestinal medical system and other various organs. Parents should understand which allergens the child is exposed to and manage the patient accurately. Drug therapy can also be selectively performed based on what kind of immune factors are causing the allergy. In general, the difference in symptoms compared to adults is that it is weak, but coughing is worse than adults. After diagnosis, living environment improvement counseling is the most important treatment.

When infants and children suffer from allergy cough, it can be easily overlooked because they are likely to have rashes, crusty scalps, or frequent colds. In addition, children's respiratory tracts are not fully developed, so they may suffer from infectious diseases several times in a year. In acute inflamed infectious diseases, cilia cells that are in charge of mucus transport stop working only for a short time, but in the body of children who have a lot of allergens, coughing, a defensive mechanism for mucus transport, can be caused. It is important to pay attention if your child is active in the area of the bedding, walks a small amount of stairs or up an uphill due to cold weather temporarily, vomits when coughing hard, makes a bell-like sound when coughing, or if your child has a runny nose and a persistent cough for a long time.

8.2. Allergy Cough in Adults

Symptom persistence and impairment with cough impact patients' daily life in most adults, and they arrive at seeking healthcare services, many of whom believe the coughing has occupied their lives. Cough and allergy care should be medically managed in a similar manner, in both children and adults, with specific focus on addressing the cause. As both singular and multiple allergic agents can provoke cough, patient involvement is greatly encouraged as the specific measures to avoid further exposure to or to limit the allergen exposure so as to decrease symptoms. From a therapeutic viewpoint, it is necessary to prescribe the ideal dosage of histamine antagonists and/or intranasal glucocorticosteroids, including many safe options for the treatment of seasonal and year-round cough sufferers with relatively minimal secondary contralateral effects. Due to this reason, when it comes to convincing adults to try an anti-allergy cough therapy, how effective it is, it is more critical for individuals to be aware of the evidence. To get a greater effect, sufferers need to adhere to their prescribed treatment programs, which may need to be supplemented with symptom relief. In order to clarify the possible dangers that their taste may impose on their unborn babies, pregnant or lactating females should keep their healthcare physicians abreast of the latest information in the field of allergen avoidance, for it helps to avoid the symptoms of inducing or worsening of obstructive breathing conditions.

Due to the fact that allergy and associated chronic coughing usually affect adults, how to appropriately diagnose and manage allergy cough in pregnant or lactating women is of much significance. Due in sizable part to these adults should have been brought about by higher levels of timely diagnosis and appropriate intervention, with the intention that the healthcare provider can tend to each patient as an individual and target the cause of his/her cough, by assessing lifestyles, exposures, and patient preferences. Notably, there exists a paucity of data addressing allergy cough treatment guidelines in older adult populations. Differences in lung function and comorbidities must also be taken into consideration when managing these patients. Elderly adults may have differing comorbidities (i.e., cardiovascular disease, diabetes, morbid obesity) that can complicate the diagnosis and management of allergy cough.

8.3. Elderly Individuals with Allergy-Induced Cough

Also, decreased mucociliary clearance, reduced compensatory respiratory effort, reduced gas exchange, and reduced cough frequency are among the conditions to be taken into account in elderly individuals with atrophic mucosa and/or reduced glandular mucus production. Impaired cough reflex, poor postnasal drainage, inability to expectorate, reduced respiratory muscle strength, and increased lung stiffness are a few examples of the reduced mucociliary clearance process. The atrophic mucosa and atrophy of secretory glands, as well as the thickening of the submucosa with consequent collapse of the nasal valve, lead to a deficiency in the diffusion of the mucociliary clearance and represent a very concentrated transudate with a high concentration of prostaglandins, which penetrates the mucosa producing irritation of nociceptive afferents. Moreover, these patients are frequently self-medicated with specific treatment for pediatric indications. Residence in the elderly, where the incidence of multiple comorbidities (gastroesophageal reflux disease, chronic obstructive pulmonary disease, asthma, postnasal drip) is very high. The use of cough-inducing substances and poor compliance further increases the complexity of the respiratory evaluation.

Many elderly individuals experience allergy-induced cough. Managing this condition in the elderly can be quite challenging due to a higher number of comorbidities, drug interactions, and age-related side effects that could further compromise these patients. Polypharmacy and poor treatment compliance can exacerbate an already complicated clinical picture. Several respiratory effects frequently associated with aging may worsen the quality of life of these individuals.

9. Complications and Risks Associated with Untreated Allergy Cough

Go to a healthcare provider if you have symptoms. When left untreated, most cases of cough will go away on their own after a few weeks. Falls can make coughs worse, so treatment may be needed so that coughs do not become severe. If a bacterial lung infection is untreated, it can lead to severe complications such as pneumonia or abscess. A healthcare specialist is likely to treat the underlying cause of the cough in most cases of cough. This could be in the form of medication or general lifestyle, environmental, or dietary modifications. The steps listed above can be used in adults and children to relieve a recurring cough. Discuss with your healthcare provider the best treatment for you based on the cause of the cough.

To avoid a chronic cough, make sure to explore your treatment options. If your cough is due to asthma, acid reflux, or a chronic lung problem, be aware that it may not resolve right away. It is incredibly rare for a regular cough from these issues to resolve without treatment. The prognosis for those who seek treatment is excellent. With a comprehensive plan that includes dietary modifications, medications, and lifestyle changes, the majority of people are able to manage their recurrent coughs. Practice good hand hygiene, maintain a healthy diet, and avoid allergens such as smoke or excessive pollution.

If your allergy-induced cough goes untreated, you could face complications and risks, including bronchitis, ear infection, sinusitis, and an inability to sleep, breathe, or concentrate. To prevent these issues from developing or worsening, treat the cause of your cough promptly. Consult your healthcare provider for an accurate diagnosis and timely treatment. The first step when it comes to treatment is to avoid allergens that cause symptoms. This could involve cleaning your environment, removing any irritants that are a trigger, or relocating to an area with fewer allergens. Everyone is different, so your healthcare provider may have other recommendations.

10. Impact of Allergy Cough on Quality of Life

For those with asthma, cough can lead to decreasing lung function with a resultant increase in overall morbidity and mortality. Allergic children may be more likely to develop poorer lung function as they continue to mature, and their frequent cough becomes a predictor of adult-onset asthma. Cough in isolation is not considered to cause pathogenesis, but emerging research suggests that cough can contribute to a person's emotional distress and decrease sleep quality and mainly decrease quality of life. Immediate caregiver quality of life (QoL) was shown to improve after treatment. This illustrates the potential high personal and financial cost for families treating a child with cough. For these reasons, ensuring ongoing child and family education is important as chronic cough can pose a long-term cost.

The repercussions of living with cough extend beyond the physical domain and can disrupt relationships and routine, limit social activities, and negatively affect a person's financial position. Some of the potential impacts are listed below: - Children can miss more days of school. - The need to take more medication can have a financial burden.

The impact of cough in allergic people can extend into the physical, social, and emotional aspects of their lives, and this can have practical implications. In the physical domain, the symptoms have the potential to cause sleep disturbance, fatigue, breathlessness, dizziness, bradycardia, vomiting, incontinence, and/or rib discomfort due to vigorous coughing. Daytime somnolence can exacerbate with cough frequency and severity and can interfere with activities of daily living and result in work and/or school absenteeism.

11. Latest Research and Innovations in Allergy Cough Treatment

Several classes of novel antitussive medications have been evaluated in chronic cough, including macrolide antibiotics, inhibitors of neurokinin receptors, cysteinyl leukotrienes, the P2X3 adenosine triphosphate receptor, transient receptor potential vanilloid subfamily 1 or S1 agonists (TRPVA1), the protease-activated receptor-2 inhibitors mepolizumab, benralizumab, and the approved PAR-2, inhalants, and the H4-antihistamine receptor peposertib (JNJ-47117096) alone and in sequence. In allergic cough, CCR3 receptor antagonists, which are eosinophil-chemotactic agents, have been evaluated as antitussives. In addition, anti-IL-5 and anti-IL-13 biologicals produce significant resolution of chronic cough in asthmatic patients. Several treatments have been tested, including induced sputum clinical drugs that are often prematurely stopped due to an adverse event, allopurinol, and nonpharmacologic options such as music therapy. Only mepolizumab, benralizumab, dupilumab, bronchial thermoplasty, specific triggers such as ACE, gastroesophageal fluids, and cardioselective beta-blockers are currently widely used in clinical practice.

The management of patients with chronic cough caused by environmental allergens and viral infections has remained largely unchanged over the last two decades due to the lack of effective medications approved by regulatory bodies. Chronic cough can be resistant to therapeutic interventions, and there is an unmet need for new antitussive agents. However, we are now at a tipping point, with several innovative new therapies poised to change the paradigm of antitussive medications for these subjects.

Allergy-proof environment. 1. Clinical prospects on allergy cough. Front. Immunol., 12:2389 2. Tackling an unmet need in allergy-associated cough: Advances in cough physiology and pathobiology. J Allergy Clin Immunol. In Practice, In Press 3. Treatment aspect of allergic cough. World Allergy Organization Journal, 15(1):100147.

The latest in allergy cough treatments Allergy cough treatment undergoing groundbreaking changes. Treatment options for allergy cough can be limited, but endota has been conducting a clinical research trial completed in 2021, one of the most recent trials to study a promising therapy. Keep reading to learn about this treatment and others that are promising to change the allergy cough paradigm.

12. Conclusion and Key Takeaways

The main takeaways from the comprehensive and detailed discussions in the previous sections are varied: For one, the presence of cough along with other symptoms can help differentiate between allergic rhinitis and chronic rhinosinusitis. Additionally, if we can distinguish between the type of cough, we can get close to the allergen or molecular mechanism that is triggering the cough. By locating the allergic allergen, we could then move to an allergist who not only can confirm the allergy with skin tests and other diagnosis, but also have a closer test for allergic lower-airways and for upper airways and a condition of hypersensitivity, the allergist could dot a confirmed diagnosis and closer treatment.

In this guide, we have answered many commonly asked questions, described symptoms, discussed allergies causing coughing, outlined treatment methods, and discussed other helpful information related to allergy cough. There is a wide range of allergies that can lead to coughing. While infectious diseases, inflammation, COPD, asthma, complications of medications, or damage done due to inhaled pollutants, to name a few, could be the primary reason for persistent, acute, or chronic cough, the allergy could be another overlooked reason for cough. Infections, flu, viruses, rhinoviruses, coronaviruses among many others may be a primary cause of cough!

Allergic cough could result from a wide range of allergens and develop into chronic or long-term conditions. It could lead to various issues such as interrupted sleep, cough syncope, urinary incontinence, or cough-induced fractures of ribs, diaphragm, or organs. While the main disease may have similar symptoms, it is essential to distinguish the primary disease from an allergic origin to manage allergic conditions effectively. The treatment options vary from decontaminating the air, reducing the perpetuation of cough, or anti-cough, anti-cholinergic, or neuro-modulated drugs. Since the risk of sophisticated allergies and complications are high in the long-term and chronic duration, it is also viable to consider consultation from a specialist in pulmonary and allergy medicine.

Conclusion

Understanding and Managing Allergy-Related Coughs

1. Introduction to Allergy-Related Coughs

A generic mechanism common to all forms of allergic nonproductive cough is the release of pre-formed histamine from degranulating mast cells, and tryptase and eosinophil cationic protein from eosinophils, damages the capillary networks that underlie the sensory airway nerves. The allergic mediators such as histamine and cysteinyl leukotriene released from multi-sensory nerve endings by capsaicin or allergen rapidly produce cough. These allergic mediators may be involved in the allergic cough reflex and the non-invasive method for measuring these mediators or exhaled nitric oxide is helpful to diagnose the allergic cause of a nonproductive cough. However, factors such as the concentration and density of the allergen, allergic status and genetic variation of the exposed subject, coexisting infection, physical activity, psychological status, seasonal variation, and general immune status may determine individual susceptibility to allergy-related cough.

Allergy-related coughs are a common presentation in both primary and tertiary care management. It is essential to understand and manage these conditions. At present, the term "cough-variant asthma" has been abandoned and lack of postnasal drip is considered as a diagnostic criterion. The occurrence of allergy-related coughs in an individual is a public health problem caused by indoor and outdoor allergens exposure. It impacts the individual's social life, sleep, and daytime activity. Even though it is not associated with increased mortality, it may be associated with complications such as syncope, physical injury-related accidents, anxiety, depression, brain injury due to hypoxemia, esophageal injury, or urinary incontinence from hyperventilation. However, there are many uncertainties regarding allergy-related coughs, such as a solvent-threshold issue, and it often goes undiagnosed. Therefore, it is common for physicians to confront a patient with a cough.

2. Causes and Triggers of Allergy-Related Coughs

One of the most common triggers of allergen-related coughing is pollen. While different types of pollen can stimulate people living in different areas, the symptoms are generally similar. They experience coughing, wheezing, and shortness of breath. People who are allergic to dogs, cats, rodents, and other furry pets will react to the dander they naturally shed. Ingesting mites is a significant problem for numerous people, and while a few species are readily visible to the naked eye, some folks develop an allergic reaction to a species that cannot be seen without a microscope. Another allergen that is present in large amounts in most households is mold. Asthma and allergy patients should pay special attention to indoor air quality, as studies have shown that air pollution can contribute to, trigger, or even aggravate respiratory allergies and asthma. In addition to smog, wood smoke, vehicle exhausts, and tobacco smoke all contain several kinds of particulate matter and gases that can cause a problem.

Allergies can be the cause of a number of symptoms, and coughing is one of the most common. Allergies stimulate the secretion of special chemicals called "histamines." The histamines set off a cascade of reactions that can lead to uncomfortable symptoms including coughing, sneezing, and a stuffy or runny nose. Allergy-related coughing can be at the very least extremely irritating, and at its worst, can be physically and emotionally draining. This can result in exhaustion, malaise, bad moods, and lower quality of life. By examining some of the allergens and other factors that stimulate coughing, we can gain insights into the potential causes of our coughing and how we can remedy our coughs.

3. Symptoms and Characteristics of Allergy-Related Coughs

Conjunctival itching, a runny nose, and sneezing are all classic hay fever symptoms. In some cases, coughing might be one of the only symptoms of hay fever during the pollen season. This is referred to as allergic rhinitis with cough. Some people may initially develop asthma, with coughing (nasal symptoms and sneezing common as well). There is a cough with this. In other words, rhinitis or upper airway inflammation normally precedes coughing in people who develop cough. While a cough and allergic rhinitis are frequently related, there are some who cough in response to allergen exposure in the absence of other typical hay fever symptoms. Even if these symptoms are minor, avoidance of offending indoor allergens may help lower cough severity. Cough and allergic rhinitis do not appear to have a significant association with one another. Wheezing, chest tightness, and coughing are the three hallmark signs of asthma, a persistent condition that makes it difficult for you to breathe.

Do you have a dry, persistent cough that gets worse at certain times of year? You may have an allergy-related cough or what healthcare professionals call allergic rhinitis with cough. The other symptoms of allergic rhinitis, such as an itchy nose, sneezing, and stuffy nose, may be mild or not present. An allergy-related cough can be a sign of hay fever. However, a pollen count or worsening of other typical hay fever symptoms may be absent. Foreign items such as mold, dust mites, and animal dander are examples of indoor and outdoor allergens that can produce allergic rhinitis with cough.

4. Diagnosis and Differential Diagnosis of Allergy-Related Coughs

Healthcare providers can diagnose atypical allergic coughs using a methacholine test, a histamine inhalation test, or a treadmill exercise test in patients with normal spirograms excluding airway hyperresponsiveness in cases with a normal spirogram and no apparent signs or respiratory sounds of asthma.

When an allergen-induced cough is suspected, healthcare providers may inquire into, or perform, some additional tests. The most important of these tests is a skin allergy test. Low serum allergen-specific IgE and a skin allergy test that is less than 3 mm in diameter has, however, been reported to have a low allergy rate. The skin allergy test has little value if the patient is taking antihistamines or corticosteroids. The cutoff of specific IgE level has not yet been established by the age of the patient or age groups.

In a thorough history, healthcare providers first obtain an overall understanding of the entire course of the disease, including the age of cough onset, potential precipitating factors, duration of cough after onset, cough interval and pattern, and cough improvement or exacerbation. The items that can help identify allergen-related cough include cough timed in sequential order and a history of symptoms associated with asthma. In elderly patients, a history of bronchial asthma is associated with allergic cough.

To diagnose allergy-related coughs, healthcare providers must listen to detailed descriptions of the cough from all concerned parties to determine if it is related to allergen exposure. The main identifying feature of cough caused by allergy is that coughing worsens when exposed to environmental factors to which the patient is allergic.

Diagnosis and Differential Diagnosis of Allergy-Related Coughs

The 'topic' for the text: Understanding and Managing Allergy-Related Coughs

5. Treatment Options for Allergy-Related Coughs

Natural remedies, such as herbal teas with honey and ingesting a bit of ginger root every day, may help alleviate allergy-related coughs. Using cool-mist humidifiers and vaporizers can instill a healthy level of moisture into the air, aiding in the thinning of mucus in the nose. As a result, allergic symptoms can be much easier to overcome. Finally, saline nasal irrigations have achieved excellent results in lessening cough-related symptoms. Similar to steam, saline irrigation can hydrate the nasal cavities and support nasal function. Garlic and turmeric are two herbs which can be used to open up the passageways, curbing mucus production and combating allergies by virtue of their antibacterial capabilities. One cannot overemphasize the importance of seeking advice from a physician or pharmacist in order to identify the most effective method for alleviating the symptoms of cough.

Common treatment options for allergy-related cough involve the use of some kind of medication. Among the over-the-counter options, antihistamines are some of the most frequently used medications that can reduce mucus production and prevent sneezing and runny nose. Decongestants can be useful as well. They can narrow blood vessels, alleviating congestion, thus making it easier to breathe. Some of them may contain pseudoephedrine, which can also be used for reducing postnasal drip and coughing. Nasal corticosteroids can reduce inflammation and stifle allergic symptoms. Prescription-strength antihistamines and decongestants might be used as well. Finally, antitussive agents can be used to soothe the throat and suppress coughing, making them highly useful for alleviating nighttime coughing.

5.1. Over-the-Counter Medications

Staying Well Hydrated. Drinking water helps to thin the mucus that lines the airway and reduce the thickness of the mucus. Tipping the head downward while drinking fluids allows the fluids to move to a part of the throat that triggers a cough less than other areas in the throat do.

Cough Suppressants. OTC cough remedies are generally not as effective as prescription cough medications. OTC medications that contain an ingredient known to suppress the cough caused by environmental substances include: Dextromethorphan, Levodropropizine.

Decongestants. Oral and nasal decongestants can help reverse a stuffy nose from an allergic reaction, which includes a runny, itchy, and sneezy nose; if a first-generation antihistamine is used, it may also help to reverse a stuffy nose if one is present. Decongestants can make it difficult to sleep and may raise a person's heart rate and blood pressure. Be sure to check with a healthcare provider before using, especially if one has underlying high blood pressure, heart disease, or prostate symptoms. A combination medication that contains a first-generation antihistamine and decongestant together, and may offer relief with longer rest due to its drowsiness properties, is also available OTC: Brompheniramine-pseudoephedrine (such as Anaplex).

Antihistamines. Over-the-counter (OTC) remedies that block the release of histamine may prevent worsening of the cough due to an allergic reaction; people with allergies often have itchy eyes, a runny or congested nose, sneezing, and itchy or runny nose. Some people make less naturally produced antihistamines for various reasons, such as aging, and may benefit more from the use of antihistamines in treating an allergy-related chronic cough. Potential side effects include mild sedation and some drying effects, such as drying of the mucus lining the lungs. Also, many over-the-counter (OTC) cold and flu medications contain antihistamines. A variety of antihistamines are available OTC, including: Diphenhydramine, Cetirizine, Loratadine, Fexofenadine.

5.2. Prescription Medications

Nasal corticosteroids are the preferred prescription medication. They work by coating the inside of the nasal passages to reduce swelling of the blood vessels. This means that there is more room for air to pass through the nasal passages, lessening the amount of air that has to travel through the back of the throat and cause coughing. The body can also specifically recruit eosinophils when it is allergic to an inhaled particle. This is what makes the eosinophil level rise in the sputum and blood of those with allergic asthma. Leukotriene modifiers are another class of medications. These are used in the long-term treatment of asthma. However, one drug in this class, montelukast (Singulair), is also approved at select dosages for management of allergic rhinitis. Similar to antihistamines, leukotriene modifiers can be appealing for patients with allergies and related cough because they also relieve sneezing and a runny nose.

Typically, a corticosteroid nasal spray is the first choice for managing cough when there are allergy symptoms present. Most corticosteroid nasal sprays are only available by prescription, but one is available over the counter: Nasacort. Nasal sprays are used by spraying the product into the nose. Some need to be sniffed in while others just need to be sprayed into the nostril. Ensuring that the patient can use the product correctly is essential in optimizing its effect. Leukotriene modifiers are other options that are only available by prescription.

5.3. Natural Remedies and Home Treatments

The goals of these treatments are to improve hydration in the nasal passages, reduce inflammation and remove mucus, and directly reduce irritation in the airways. Caffeine and some diuretics that induce drinking more fluids are well-known cough reducers and can increase nasal and airway moisture content. Potentially useful dietary changes include consuming foods with an inflammatory component, often omega-3 polyunsaturated fatty acids, or an increase in the content of antioxidants. Patients may benefit from foods containing natural antioxidants such as citrus and berries, nuts and seeds, fruits and vegetables, green, red, and orange peppers, spinach, sweet potatoes, and whole grains. Butterbur, also known as Petasites officinalis, is an herb that some practitioners believe can combat cough and pre-empt histamine release when taken before an allergic event. Patients should exercise caution with butterbur and avoid butterbur products with hepatotoxic substances called pyrrolizidine alkaloids (PAs).

Because many prescription and over-the-counter remedies can treat allergy-related coughs, it can be useful to consider home-based and alternative therapies. Further, some of these approaches can be adopted in combination with pharmacologic treatments. Non-pharmacological interventions used to treat coughs related to established allergic diseases often target nasal symptoms, asthma, or allergic rhinitis. For example, therapies that increase the moisture content of inspired air, improve indoor air quality, and humidify the environment generally alleviate coughing and other symptoms of allergic reaction. Some specific therapies include saline nasal irrigation, steam inhalation, which should not be employed in a small enclosed space with incredibly hot steam, local increases in airway humidity, dietary changes and caffeine, air filtration, and less often, herbal remedies such as butterbur.

6. Preventive Strategies for Allergy-Related Coughs

Allergy-proofing your home can be helpful in reducing the incidence of associated allergic coughs. Using a dehumidifier to lower indoor humidity, allergen-free pillows and mattresses, and a high-efficiency particulate air (HEPA) filter can help prevent exposure to dust mites. Vacuuming, using protectors on mattresses and pillows, and frequent dusting can help remove these allergens from your home. Individuals should promote a healthy bedroom environment by keeping their windows closed when the pollen count is high and dusting and vacuuming frequently. Parents may want to use anti-allergy mattress covers for a child's bedding to reduce exposure. In general, patients should limit indoor and outdoor exposure during times when they know the allergen counts will be high, or when the allergen itself is high.

To avoid having allergy-related coughs, individuals can take some preventive measures to either reduce the chances of having an allergic reaction or avoid known allergens. Preventive strategies include allergy-proofing homes, checking the local pollen forecast before outdoor activities, and covering one's nose with a mask when exposed to allergens like dust, mold, and pollen. Individuals concerned with allergic reactions to chemicals may want to use natural cleaners and detergents at home. Individuals with allergies to food should check ingredient labels on food products to ensure they do not contain triggers. Some people may want to consider decreasing meat in their diet because meats, particularly beef, are a known source of allergic coughs.

6.1. Avoiding Allergens

For those repeatedly affected, it is beneficial to combine both quick relief and preventive medications with allergen avoidance. While irritants and pollutants are generally easier to avoid than allergens, avoiding irritants and pollution can also provide a great deal of benefit during periods of repeated CVA.

The best evidence to support lifestyle changes is when allergies are a trigger. The substances that occasionally cause coughs are often difficult to avoid. For example, benign particles such as dust, mold, and pollen are difficult to keep out of the air we breathe, although different measures can help keep us exposed to them to a minimum, particularly inside buildings. While there is certainly nothing wrong with open windows, allergies are more easily managed when filtered air is brought into our living environment through the use of air purifiers with HEPA filters or airtight air conditioning. It is also beneficial to clean living spaces thoroughly once a week, performing the larger cleaning tasks less frequently, and targeting areas where mold and dust can collect. Examples of this could include that old bank of mail, underneath the carpet, inside air ducts, and on the premises of any pets as well as in rooms with returning indoor plants. It helps those around us to know allergen-reducing strategies for any outside property, including when to keep windows closed during high grass pollen counts, planting pollen-free gardens, smoking bans on the property and nearby, and so forth.

6.2. Allergy-Proofing Your Home

Keep all surfaces like window blinds, countertops, and ceiling fan blades clean and dry. Regular cleaning for dust and pet dander involves more than just removing the little particles from visible surfaces. If you suspect dust mites are affecting allergies, vacuum the mattress and box spring to remove possible allergens and consider using zippered casings. When cleaning items with removable filters, such as room air purifiers, follow the instructions for disposal. To keep pet allergens to a minimum, bathe and groom pets regularly, at least once a week. If bath time is a battle, use a professional pet groomer or pet store that offers grooming services. It doesn't matter what breed your pet is, pets with fur can still track in pollen. That's why during peak pollen times, wiping down fur protects your indoor air.

The more you can minimize allergens in your living space, the less likely an allergy-related cough will develop. Hypoallergenic pillows, mattresses, and encasements protect you from dust mites. These encasements form a barrier between the mites and you to block the allergens that these pesky bugs create. Beef up ventilation by using exhaust fans or opening windows, especially in the kitchen and bathroom. When using an air conditioner, keep the outdoor air intake closed. Change or clean heating and cooling filters once or twice per month. Dirty filters can produce a sneeze-inducing amount of dust.

6.3. Dietary Considerations

The consumption of adequate amounts of fruits and vegetables and fermented foods and a healthy diet pattern, such as the Mediterranean diet pattern, may be beneficial to reduce symptoms associated with chronic cough, although there is no good evidence in this area of work. Anecdotally, lemon juice (an organic acid found in the rind and pulp), vitamin C-rich fruits and vegetables, and anti-inflammatory and potent antioxidant-rich red and purple fruits (including berries, cherries, and fruits with similarly colored fruit flesh) have been purported to improve chronic cough. Unlike in asthma, increased sodium intake is not known to increase dilution of secretions in the airways or sputum production in patients with chronic cough; therefore, excessive salt intake will not lead to excessive bronchial and cough reflex activation. However, this consideration needs to be balanced with known negative health consequences of excessive salt intake, which is the likely root cause of this suggestion.

In some patients, dietary factors may potentially contribute to managing or treating the cough-elaborating signals, eighth cranial nerve, and cough receptor via the mechanisms described earlier. Although not at the forefront of patient management, one recognized association is between citric acid and cough, more commonly through reflux esophagitis and cough, although this has been proposed as a cofactor or a trigger for airway citric acid-elicited cough. Another is the cough-eliciting action of capsaicin in chili and spicy food, a hallmark of which is the pungency and recognizable irritant action of chili-containing foods. Limited trials of low histamine-rich foods and hypoglycemic diets are reported anecdotally.

7. When to Seek Medical Attention for Allergy-Related Coughs

A respiratory infection due to a virus (cold or flu) can be a cause. This is more likely to be at play if an itchy throat is accompanied by sneezing, a runny nose, a cough, or a scratchy feeling in the eyes. It can take a cough four weeks to resolve after a viral infection, such as the flu. Since the throat gets irritated over time and a person starts coughing, the diagnosis is usually either postnasal drip or asthma. Sinusitis can begin to occur if untreated. Postnasal flow can be caused by untreated sinusitis. All of these indications can be present. If a person's coughing becomes more frequent than normal for him or her, or if he or she has more shortness of breath than usual, they should have these symptoms assessed. This type of a cough can also occur as a result of other circumstances. When a person either wheezes when he breathes or experiences more nasal congestion when he lies down or lies on one's side, he or she can get evaluated for asthma. Asthma can be caused by allergies.

Allergies can make people cough for a number of reasons. In some cases, they cough because pollen or other allergens irritate the lining of the nose or throat. Getting away from allergens and taking medicine as directed can help with these types of coughs to help you feel better fast.

8. Emergency Care for Severe Allergic Reactions

Emergency antigen-specific therapy includes: • Epinephrine: Use the dose of epinephrine Auto-Injector 0.01mg/kg up to 0.3 mg in children and 0.3 to 0.5 mg in adolescents who are severely wheezing or have a marginally life-threatening allergic reaction within the first 5 minutes, and then repeat the dose every 3-5 minutes. • Inj. Adrenaline/Epinephrine 1mg/ml IV or 0.01mg/kg • IV bolus up to 0.1 mg per dose at a time; may be repeated every 5 minutes for 2 doses or Tab. Actrapid/Insulin (IV) Bolus, IV Dilution 50ml Dusk in NS 30ml & Draw 1.5ml in 10ml Syringe, Discard 6.5ml D/W- Prepared solution? 3mg, the solution may be given either IV as a bolus or subcutaneous or IM. • Care should be taken while administering vasopressors and other vaso-actives in patients known to have RT with a. Epinephrine: 0.01 mg/kg up to a dose of 0.3-0.5 mg, given at a rate of 0.3 mg/kg per minute, the patient must be in a supine position, and the drugs are prepared in a dilution. • If possible, lie the patient in a supine position when adrenaline is given in the form of intracutaneous or subcutaneous. When???? positional n. B. IV bolus Adrenaline may be given with an antihistamine like ranitidine (Zintec) processing, very true.

GE Care for severe allergic reactions includes: • Severe coughing/wheezing/respiratory distress • Difficult or noisy breathing/turning blue/unconsciousness • Swollen

tongue with difficulty breathing • Change in voice •
Wheezing/unspecified stridor